STOMACH ULCER DIET COOKBOOK FOR SENIORS

Nutritious Anti-Inflammatory Recipes Designed To Naturally Manage Gastric Ulcer and Fortify Digestive Systems

Emily O. Wells

Introduction:

In the context of digestive health, stomach ulcers stand as a significant concern, particularly among seniors. The delicate balance of the digestive system can be disrupted by various factors, leading to the development of ulcers in the stomach lining. As we age, the likelihood of encountering such issues increases, making it imperative for seniors to understand how to manage and alleviate the symptoms associated with stomach ulcers.

Hence, this cookbook aims to provide seniors with a deeper understanding of stomach ulcers and equip them with practical knowledge to navigate their dietary choices effectively. By embracing a diet specifically designed to support digestive health, seniors can alleviate discomfort, promote healing, and enhance their overall well-being.

Jude's Transformation Journey with Stomach Ulcers

Jude had struggled for years with stomach ulcers, feeling frustrated and limited by his condition. Then, he stumbled upon a stomach ulcer diet cookbook specifically designed for seniors like him. With its guidance, he discovered a world of flavorful and healing recipes tailored to soothe his stomach and nourish his body.

He found relief in the carefully crafted meal plans and the wealth of information on managing stomach ulcers. He learned to make healthier choices at restaurants, manage portion sizes, and communicate his dietary needs effectively.

With each meal he prepared from this cookbook, Jude felt a renewed sense of hope and empowerment. Gone were the days of bland and boring meals—he now enjoyed delicious dishes that not only satisfied his taste buds but also supported his digestive health.

Thanks to this cookbook, Jude's journey with stomach ulcers transformed from one of struggle to one of empowerment. He embraced his new culinary adventures with enthusiasm, grateful for the newfound freedom and vitality it brought to his life.

TABLE OF CONTENT

CHAPTER 1

UNDERSTANDING STOMACH ULCERS

Stomach ulcers, also known as **gastric ulcers** or **peptic ulcers**, are open sores that develop on the lining of the stomach. These ulcers can cause varying degrees of discomfort and pain, ranging from mild to severe. Understanding the nature of stomach ulcers is essential for seniors to effectively manage their condition and maintain optimal health.

What are Stomach Ulcers?

Stomach ulcers occur when the protective lining of the stomach becomes damaged, allowing digestive acids to erode the underlying tissue. This erosion leads to the formation of open sores or ulcers, which can result in symptoms such as abdominal pain, bloating, nausea, and indigestion. Stomach ulcers can also lead to more serious complications if left untreated, including bleeding or perforation of the stomach lining.

Causes and Risk Factors

Several factors contribute to the development of stomach ulcers, including:

1. **Infection with Helicobacter pylori (H. pylori) bacteria:** This bacterium is a common cause of stomach ulcers and can be transmitted through contaminated food or water.

2. **Non-steroidal anti-inflammatory drugs (NSAIDs):** Long-term use of NSAIDs such as aspirin, ibuprofen, and naproxen can irritate the stomach lining and increase the risk of developing ulcers.

3. **Excessive alcohol consumption:** Alcohol can irritate the stomach lining and contribute to the formation of ulcers, particularly in individuals who consume alcohol regularly or in large quantities.

4. **Smoking:** Smoking can weaken the stomach's protective barrier and impair its ability to heal, making smokers more susceptible to developing ulcers.

5. **Stress:** While stress alone does not cause ulcers, it can exacerbate existing symptoms and increase the likelihood of complications.

Symptoms and Diagnosis

The symptoms of stomach ulcers can vary depending on the severity of the condition. Common symptoms include:

- Abdominal pain or discomfort, which may be dull, burning, or gnawing in nature
- Bloating or fullness, particularly after meals
- Nausea or vomiting
- Loss of appetite or weight loss
- Dark, tarry stools (indicating bleeding)
- Difficulty swallowing or frequent belching

Diagnosing stomach ulcers typically involves a combination of medical history review, physical examination, and diagnostic tests such as:

1. **Upper endoscopy:** A procedure in which a thin, flexible tube with a camera (endoscope) is inserted through the mouth and into the stomach to visualize the ulcer and obtain tissue samples for biopsy.
2. **Barium swallow or upper gastrointestinal series:** X-ray imaging of the upper digestive tract after swallowing a contrast dye (barium) to highlight any abnormalities in the stomach or esophagus.
3. **Blood, stool, or breath tests:** These tests may be used to detect the presence of H. pylori infection or assess for signs of bleeding or inflammation.

Treatment Options

The treatment of stomach ulcers typically involves a combination of medication, lifestyle modifications, and dietary changes. Common treatment options include:

1. **Proton pump inhibitors (PPIs) or H2-receptor antagonists:** These medications reduce the production of stomach acid, helping to heal ulcers and alleviate symptoms.

2. **Antibiotics:** If H. pylori infection is present, a course of antibiotics may be prescribed to eradicate the bacteria and prevent recurrence of ulcers.

3. **Antacids:** Over-the-counter antacids can provide temporary relief from symptoms by neutralizing stomach acid and soothing irritation.

4. **Lifestyle modifications:** Seniors with stomach ulcers are often advised to avoid smoking, limit alcohol consumption, and manage stress to reduce symptoms and promote healing.

5. **Dietary changes:** Certain foods and beverages can exacerbate symptoms of stomach ulcers, while others may help soothe inflammation and support healing. Adopting a stomach ulcer-friendly diet can play a crucial role in managing the condition and preventing recurrence.

CHAPTER 2:

THE IMPORTANCE OF DIET IN MANAGING STOMACH ULCERS

Diet plays a pivotal role in managing stomach ulcers, as certain foods can either exacerbate symptoms or promote healing and symptom relief. Seniors with stomach ulcers must pay careful attention to their dietary choices to alleviate discomfort, support healing, and prevent recurrence of ulcers. This chapter explores how diet affects stomach ulcers, provides guidance on foods to avoid and include, and discusses the importance of meal timing and portion control in managing this condition.

How Diet Affects Stomach Ulcers

The foods and beverages consumed can significantly impact the development and severity of stomach ulcers. Certain dietary factors can exacerbate symptoms and irritate the stomach lining, while others can help soothe inflammation and promote healing.

Foods to Avoid

Seniors with stomach ulcers should avoid or reduce the intake of the following foods and beverages:

1. Spicy and acidic foods: Foods high in spice, such as chili peppers and hot sauces, can irritate the stomach lining and exacerbate symptoms. Acidic foods and beverages, such as citrus fruits, tomatoes, and coffee, can also increase stomach acid production and worsen ulcers.

2. Fatty and fried foods: High-fat and fried foods can delay stomach emptying and increase the risk of acid reflux, leading to discomfort and exacerbation of symptoms.

3. Carbonated beverages: Carbonated drinks, including soda and sparkling water, can increase gas production and contribute to bloating and discomfort.

4. Alcohol: Alcohol can irritate the stomach lining and increase the risk of developing ulcers, making it advisable for seniors with stomach ulcers to limit or avoid alcohol consumption.

5. Caffeine: Caffeinated beverages such as coffee, tea, and energy drinks can stimulate acid production in the stomach and exacerbate symptoms of ulcers.

6. Spicy condiments and sauces: Condiments such as hot sauce, salsa, and mustard can irritate the stomach lining and trigger symptoms in individuals with stomach ulcers.

7. Processed and high-sodium foods: Processed foods high in salt and preservatives can irritate the stomach lining and exacerbate inflammation, making them best avoided by seniors with stomach ulcers.

Foods to Include

On the other hand, incorporating the following foods into the diet can help soothe inflammation, promote healing, and alleviate symptoms of stomach ulcers:

1. High-fiber foods: Fiber-rich foods such as fruits, vegetables, whole grains, and legumes can help regulate digestion, prevent constipation, and promote overall digestive health.

2. Lean proteins: Lean sources of protein, such as poultry, fish, tofu, and legumes, are easier to

digest and less likely to irritate the stomach lining compared to fatty meats.

3. Non-acidic fruits: Seniors with stomach ulcers can enjoy non-acidic fruits such as bananas, apples, melons, and pears, which are gentle on the stomach and provide essential nutrients and antioxidants.

4. Vegetables: Cooked or steamed vegetables, such as carrots, spinach, squash, and sweet potatoes, are nutritious additions to the diet and can help soothe inflammation in the stomach.

5. Dairy products: Low-fat dairy products such as milk, yogurt, and cheese can provide calcium and protein without exacerbating symptoms of stomach ulcers.

6. Herbal teas: Herbal teas such as chamomile, ginger, and licorice root tea can help soothe inflammation, alleviate discomfort, and promote relaxation in individuals with stomach ulcers.

7. Healthy fats: Incorporating sources of healthy fats, such as avocados, nuts, seeds, and olive oil, can provide essential nutrients and promote satiety without aggravating stomach ulcers.

Meal Timing and Portion Control

Whilst choosing appropriate foods, seniors with stomach ulcers should pay attention to meal timing and portion control to manage symptoms effectively:

1. Eat smaller, more frequent meals: Consuming smaller meals throughout the day can help prevent excessive stomach acid production and reduce the likelihood of discomfort and bloating.

2. Avoid late-night eating: Eating large meals or snacks close to bedtime can increase the risk of acid reflux and disrupt sleep, so seniors with stomach ulcers should aim to eat dinner at least two to three hours before bedtime.

3. Chew food thoroughly: Chewing food thoroughly aids in digestion and reduces the workload on the stomach, helping to prevent discomfort and promote efficient nutrient absorption.

4. Practice mindful eating: Paying attention to hunger and fullness cues and eating slowly can help prevent overeating and promote better digestion in seniors with stomach ulcers.

Chapter 3:

BUILDING A HEALTHY DIET PLAN

A healthy diet plan is crucial for seniors with stomach ulcers to effectively manage their condition, promote healing, and support overall well-being. However, the key components of building a balanced and nourishing diet plan includes:

Creating a Balanced Plate

A balanced plate is essential for providing the necessary nutrients while minimizing irritation to the stomach lining. Seniors with stomach ulcers should aim to include a variety of foods from different food groups to ensure adequate intake of essential nutrients. The following principles can guide the creation of a balanced plate:

1. **Fill half of your plate with fruits and vegetables:** Fruits and vegetables are rich in vitamins, minerals, and antioxidants that support digestive health and overall well-being. Choose a variety of colors

and types to maximize nutrient intake.

2. **Include lean protein sources:** Lean proteins such as poultry, fish, tofu, legumes, and eggs are essential for muscle repair and maintenance. Opt for grilled, baked, or steamed protein sources to minimize added fats and oils.

3. **Incorporate whole grains:** Whole grains such as brown rice, quinoa, oats, and whole wheat bread provide fiber, vitamins, and minerals essential for digestive health. Choose whole grains over refined grains to promote satiety and support regular bowel movements.

4. **Add healthy fats:** Healthy fats from sources such as avocados, nuts, seeds, and olive oil provide essential fatty acids and support nutrient absorption. Use small amounts of healthy fats in cooking or as toppings for salads and vegetables.

5. **Limit added sugars and processed foods:** Minimize consumption of sugary snacks, desserts, and processed foods high in refined carbohydrates, as they can exacerbate symptoms of stomach

ulcers   and   contribute   to
inflammation.

Importance of Hydration

Adequate and Proper hydration is essential for digestive health and overall well-being, especially for seniors with stomach ulcers. Adequate fluid intake helps maintain the mucous lining of the stomach, prevents constipation, and supports digestion. Seniors with stomach ulcers should aim to drink plenty of fluids throughout the day, including water, herbal teas, and diluted fruit juices. Thus, Avoiding excessive caffeine and alcohol consumption is also important, as these beverages can irritate the stomach lining and worsen symptoms.

Planning Meals and Snacks

Planning meals and snacks in advance can help seniors with stomach ulcers make healthier choices and avoid trigger foods. Consider the following strategies for meal planning:

1. Create a weekly meal plan: Plan out meals and snacks for the week, taking into account dietary preferences, nutritional needs, and any food intolerances or allergies.

2. Shop for fresh, whole foods: Stock up on fresh fruits, vegetables, lean proteins, whole grains, and healthy fats to have nutritious ingredients on hand for meals and snacks.

3. Prepare meals in advance: Batch cooking and meal prep can save time and ensure that healthy meals are readily available throughout the week. Prepare large batches of soups, stews, or grain-based salads that can be portioned out and stored for later consumption.

4. Pack portable snacks: Keep nutritious snacks on hand for times when hunger strikes between meals. Portable options such as fresh fruit, nuts, yogurt, and whole grain crackers can provide energy and satiety without aggravating stomach ulcers.

5. Listen to your body: Pay attention to hunger and fullness cues, and adjust portion sizes accordingly. Eating slowly and mindfully can help prevent overeating and promote better digestion.

Chapter 4

BREAKFAST RECIPES SUITABLE FOR SENIORS WITH STOMACH ULCERS

1. Oatmeal with Fresh Fruit

Ingredients:

- 1/2 cup old-fashioned oats
- 1 cup water or low-fat milk
- 1/2 banana, sliced
- 1/4 cup blueberries
- 1 tablespoon honey or maple syrup (optional)

Instructions:

1. In a small saucepan, bring water or milk to a boil.
2. Stir in oats and reduce heat to low. Simmer for 5-7 minutes, stirring occasionally, until oats are cooked and thickened.
3. Remove from heat and let cool slightly.
4. Top with sliced banana, blueberries, and a drizzle of honey or maple syrup if desired.
5. Serve warm.

Cooking time: 10 minutes

2. Greek Yogurt Parfait

Ingredients:

- 1/2 cup plain Greek yogurt
- 1/4 cup granola (choose low-fat, low-sugar options)
- 1/4 cup sliced strawberries
- 1 tablespoon honey or agave syrup (optional)

Instructions:

1. In a glass or bowl, layer Greek yogurt, granola, and sliced strawberries.
2. Repeat layers until ingredients are used up.
3. Drizzle with honey or agave syrup if desired.
4. Serve immediately.

Cooking time: 5 minutes

3. Whole Grain Toast with Nut Butter

Ingredients:

- 1-2 slices whole grain bread
- 1-2 tablespoons nut butter (almond, peanut, or cashew)
- 1/2 banana, sliced (optional)

Instructions:

1. Toast whole grain bread until golden brown.
2. Spread nut butter evenly on toasted bread slices.
3. Top with sliced banana if desired.
4. Serve immediately.

Cooking time: 3-5 minutes

4. Scrambled Eggs with Spinach

Ingredients:

- 2 eggs
- 1/4 cup fresh spinach, chopped
- 1 tablespoon low-fat milk (optional)
- Salt and pepper to taste

Instructions:

1. In a bowl, whisk together eggs, milk (if using), salt, and pepper until well combined.
2. Heat a non-stick skillet over medium heat.
3. Add chopped spinach to the skillet and cook until wilted, about 1-2 minutes.
4. Pour whisked eggs into the skillet and scramble until cooked through, about 2-3 minutes.
5. Serve hot.

Cooking time: 5 minutes

5. Cottage Cheese with Peach Slices

Ingredients:

- 1/2 cup low-fat cottage cheese
- 1 fresh peach, sliced
- 1 tablespoon honey or agave syrup (optional)

Instructions:

1. In a bowl, spoon cottage cheese.
2. Top with sliced peach.
3. Drizzle with honey or agave syrup if desired.
4. Serve immediately.

Cooking time: 2 minutes

6. Smoothie with Banana and Spinach

Ingredients:

- 1 ripe banana
- 1/2 cup fresh spinach
- 1/2 cup plain Greek yogurt
- 1/2 cup water or low-fat milk
- 1 tablespoon honey or maple syrup (optional)
- Ice cubes (optional)

Instructions:

- In a blender, combine banana, spinach, Greek yogurt, water or milk, and honey or maple syrup if using.
- Blend until smooth and creamy.
- Add ice cubes if desired and blend again until smooth.
- Pour into a glass and serve immediately.

Cooking time: 5 minutes

7. Mashed Avocado on Whole Grain Toast

Ingredients:

- 1 ripe avocado
- 1-2 slices whole grain bread, toasted
- Salt and pepper to taste

Instructions:

- Cut avocado in half, remove the pit, and scoop the flesh into a bowl.
- Mash avocado with a fork until smooth.
- Season with salt and pepper to taste.
- Spread mashed avocado evenly on toasted bread slices.
- Serve immediately.

Cooking time: 5 minutes

8. Rice Cake with Almond Butter and Banana Slices

Ingredients:

- 1 rice cake
- 1-2 tablespoons almond butter
- 1/2 banana, sliced

Instructions:

1. Spread almond butter evenly on the rice cake.
2. Top with sliced banana.
3. Serve immediately.

Cooking time: 2 minutes

9. Quinoa Porridge with Cinnamon and Berries

Ingredients:

- 1/2 cup cooked quinoa
- 1/4 teaspoon ground cinnamon
- 1/4 cup mixed berries (strawberries, blueberries, raspberries)
- 1 tablespoon honey or maple syrup (optional)

Instructions:

1. In a small saucepan, heat cooked quinoa with cinnamon until warmed through.
2. Transfer quinoa porridge to a bowl.
3. Top with mixed berries.
4. Drizzle with honey or maple syrup if desired.
5. Serve warm.

Cooking time: 5 minutes

10. Baked Apple with Cinnamon

Ingredients:

- 1 apple
- 1/4 teaspoon ground cinnamon
- 1 tablespoon honey or maple syrup (optional)

Instructions:

1. Preheat oven to 375°F (190°C).
2. Core the apple and slice it horizontally.
3. Place apple slices on a baking sheet lined with parchment paper.
4. Sprinkle ground cinnamon evenly over apple slices.
5. Drizzle with honey or maple syrup if desired.

6. Bake for 15-20 minutes or until apples are tender.
7. Serve warm.

Cooking time: 20 minutes

Chapter 5

LUNCH RECIPES TAILORED SPECIFICALLY FOR SENIORS WITH STOMACH ULCERS

1. Grilled Chicken and Vegetable Salad

Ingredients:

- 1 boneless, skinless chicken breast
- Mixed salad greens (spinach, lettuce, arugula)
- Assorted vegetables (bell peppers, cucumbers, tomatoes)
- Olive oil
- Lemon juice
- Salt and pepper

Instructions:

1. Preheat a grill or grill pan over medium-high heat.
2. Season the chicken breast with salt, pepper, and a drizzle of olive oil.
3. Grill the chicken for 6-8 minutes per side, or until cooked through.
4. Meanwhile, prepare the salad by washing and chopping the mixed greens and vegetables.

5. In a small bowl, whisk together olive oil, lemon juice, salt, and pepper to make the dressing.
6. Slice the grilled chicken and arrange it on top of the salad.
7. Drizzle the dressing over the salad and chicken.
8. Serve immediately.

Cooking time: 15-20 minutes

2. Quinoa and Vegetable Stir-Fry

Ingredients:

- 1 cup quinoa
- Assorted vegetables (broccoli, bell peppers, carrots, snap peas)
- Garlic, minced
- Low-sodium soy sauce
- Sesame oil
- Salt and pepper

Instructions:

1. Cook quinoa according to package instructions and set aside.
2. Heat sesame oil in a large skillet or wok over medium heat.
3. Add minced garlic and stir-fry for 1 minute.

4. Add assorted vegetables to the skillet and stir-fry until tender-crisp.
5. Stir in cooked quinoa and season with low-sodium soy sauce, salt, and pepper.
6. Cook for an additional 2-3 minutes, stirring frequently.
7. Remove from heat and serve hot.

Cooking time: 25-30 minutes

3. Turkey and Avocado Wrap

Ingredients:

- Whole grain tortillas
- Sliced turkey breast
- Ripe avocado, sliced
- Mixed salad greens
- Hummus
- Lemon juice
- Salt and pepper

Instructions:

1. Lay out a tortilla and spread a layer of hummus on it.
2. Arrange slices of turkey breast, avocado, and mixed salad greens on top.

3. Drizzle with lemon juice and season with salt and pepper.
4. Roll up the tortilla tightly, folding in the sides as you go.
5. Slice the wrap in half diagonally and serve.

Cooking time: 5-10 minutes

4. Vegetable and Lentil Soup

Ingredients:

- 1 cup dried lentils, rinsed
- Assorted vegetables (onions, carrots, celery, zucchini)
- Low-sodium vegetable broth
- Garlic, minced
- Italian seasoning
- Salt and pepper

Instructions:

1. In a large pot, sauté minced garlic in olive oil over medium heat until fragrant.
2. Add diced onions, carrots, and celery to the pot and cook until softened.
3. Stir in dried lentils, Italian seasoning, salt, and pepper.
4. Pour in vegetable broth and bring to a boil.

5. Reduce heat to low and simmer for 20-25 minutes, or until lentils are tender.
6. Add diced zucchini and continue to simmer for an additional 5 minutes.
7. Adjust seasoning to taste and serve hot.

Cooking time: 30-40 minutes

5. Salmon and Quinoa Salad

Ingredients:

- 1 salmon fillet
- Cooked quinoa
- Mixed salad greens
- Cherry tomatoes, halved
- Cucumber, sliced
- Lemon juice
- Olive oil
- Salt and pepper

Instructions:

1. Preheat the oven to 400°F (200°C).
2. Season the salmon fillet with salt, pepper, and a drizzle of olive oil.
3. Place the salmon on a baking sheet lined with parchment paper.
4. Bake for 12-15 minutes, or until the salmon is cooked through and flakes easily with a fork.

5. Meanwhile, prepare the salad by tossing mixed greens, cherry tomatoes, and cucumber in a bowl.
6. In a small bowl, whisk together lemon juice, olive oil, salt, and pepper to make the dressing.
7. Once the salmon is cooked, flake it into bite-sized pieces.
8. Divide cooked quinoa among serving plates and top with the salad mixture and flaked salmon.
9. Drizzle the dressing over the salad and serve immediately.

Cooking time: 20-25 minutes

6. Tofu and Vegetable Stir-Fry

Ingredients:

- Firm tofu, cubed
- Assorted vegetables (broccoli, bell peppers, snap peas, mushrooms)
- Garlic, minced
- Low-sodium soy sauce
- Sesame oil
- Cornstarch
- Salt and pepper

Instructions:

1. Press tofu to remove excess moisture and cut into cubes.
2. Heat sesame oil in a large skillet or wok over medium heat.
3. Add minced garlic and cubed tofu to the skillet and cook until tofu is golden brown.
4. Remove tofu from the skillet and set aside.
5. In the same skillet, stir-fry assorted vegetables until tender-crisp.
6. In a small bowl, whisk together low-sodium soy sauce, cornstarch, salt, and pepper to make the sauce.
7. Return tofu to the skillet and pour the sauce over the tofu and vegetables.
8. Cook for an additional 2-3 minutes, stirring frequently.
9. Remove from heat and serve hot.

Cooking time: 20-25 minutes

7. Egg Salad Lettuce Wraps

Ingredients:

- Hard-boiled eggs, chopped
- Greek yogurt
- Dijon mustard
- Chopped celery
- Chopped green onions
- Salt and pepper

- Butter lettuce leaves

Instructions:

1. In a mixing bowl, combine chopped hard-boiled eggs, Greek yogurt, Dijon mustard, chopped celery, and green onions.
2. Season with salt and pepper to taste and mix until well combined.
3. Spoon the egg salad mixture onto butter lettuce leaves.
4. Roll up the lettuce leaves and secure with toothpicks, if necessary.
5. Serve chilled.

Cooking time: 15-20 minutes

8. Vegetable and Bean Burrito Bowl

Ingredients:

- Cooked brown rice
- Mixed beans (black beans, kidney beans)
- Assorted vegetables (bell peppers, onions, corn)
- Salsa
- Avocado, sliced
- Fresh cilantro, chopped
- Lime wedges
- Salt and pepper

Instructions:

1. Heat a skillet over medium heat and sauté assorted vegetables until tender.
2. Warm mixed beans in a separate saucepan over low heat.
3. To assemble the burrito bowl, divide cooked brown rice among serving bowls.
4. Top with sautéed vegetables, mixed beans, salsa, sliced avocado, and chopped cilantro.
5. Squeeze fresh lime juice over the bowl and season with salt and pepper to taste.
6. Serve hot.

Cooking time: 20-25 minutes

9. Turkey and Vegetable Stir-Fry

Ingredients:

- Ground turkey
- Assorted vegetables (broccoli, carrots, bell peppers)
- Garlic, minced
- Low-sodium soy sauce
- Sesame oil
- Cornstarch
- Salt and pepper

Instructions:

1. Heat sesame oil in a large skillet or wok over medium heat.
2. Add minced garlic and ground turkey to the skillet and cook until turkey is browned.
3. Remove turkey from the skillet and set aside.
4. In the same skillet, stir-fry assorted vegetables until tender-crisp.
5. In a small bowl, whisk together low-sodium soy sauce, cornstarch, salt, and pepper to make the sauce.
6. Return turkey to the skillet and pour the sauce over the turkey and vegetables.
7. Cook for an additional 2-3 minutes, stirring frequently.
8. Remove from heat and serve hot.

Cooking time: 20-25 minutes

10. Veggie and Hummus Wrap

Ingredients:

- Whole grain tortillas
- Hummus
- Assorted vegetables (bell peppers, cucumbers, carrots, spinach)
- Sliced avocado
- Sprouts (alfalfa, broccoli, or mixed)

- Lemon juice
- Salt and pepper

Instructions:

1. Spread a layer of hummus onto a whole grain tortilla.
2. Arrange assorted vegetables, sliced avocado, and sprouts on top of the hummus.
3. Drizzle with lemon juice and season with salt and pepper.
4. Roll up the tortilla tightly, folding in the sides as you go.
5. Slice the wrap in half diagonally and serve.

Cooking time: 5-10 minutes

Chapter 6

DINNER RECIPES TAILORED FOR SENIORS WITH STOMACH ULCERS:

1. Baked Salmon with Steamed Vegetables

Ingredients:

- 4 oz salmon fillets
- 1 cup mixed vegetables (such as broccoli, carrots, and cauliflower)
- 1 tablespoon olive oil
- Salt and pepper to taste
- Lemon wedges for serving

Instructions:

1. Preheat the oven to 375°F (190°C).
2. Place the salmon fillets on a baking sheet lined with parchment paper.
3. Drizzle the salmon with olive oil and season with salt and pepper.
4. Bake the salmon in the preheated oven for 15-20 minutes, or until cooked through and flaky.
5. While the salmon is baking, steam the mixed vegetables until tender, about 7-10 minutes.
6. Serve the baked salmon with steamed vegetables and lemon wedges on the side.

Cooking Time: 25-30 minutes

Nutritional Value (per serving):

- Calories: 300
- Protein: 25g
- Carbohydrates: 10g
- Fat: 15g
- Fiber: 4g

2. Turkey Meatballs with Whole Wheat Pasta

Ingredients:

- 1 lb ground turkey
- 1/4 cup breadcrumbs
- 1 egg
- 1/4 cup grated Parmesan cheese
- 2 cups whole wheat pasta
- 1 cup marinara sauce
- 1 tablespoon olive oil
- Salt and pepper to taste
- Fresh basil leaves for garnish

Instructions:

1. In a bowl, combine ground turkey, breadcrumbs, egg, Parmesan cheese, salt, and pepper. Mix until well combined.
2. Roll the mixture into meatballs of equal size.

3. Heat olive oil in a skillet over medium heat. Add the meatballs and cook until browned on all sides and cooked through, about 10-12 minutes.
4. Meanwhile, cook the whole wheat pasta according to package instructions.
5. Heat the marinara sauce in a separate saucepan.
6. Serve the turkey meatballs over whole wheat pasta, topped with marinara sauce and fresh basil leaves.

Cooking Time: 20-25 minutes

Nutritional Value (per serving):

- Calories: 350
- Protein: 30g
- Carbohydrates: 35g
- Fat: 10g
- Fiber: 6g

3. Stir-Fried Tofu and Vegetables

Ingredients:

- 1 block firm tofu, drained and cubed
- 2 cups mixed vegetables (such as bell peppers, snap peas, and mushrooms)
- 2 tablespoons soy sauce (low-sodium)
- 1 tablespoon sesame oil
- 1 tablespoon olive oil
- 2 cloves garlic, minced

- 1 teaspoon grated ginger
- Cooked brown rice for serving
- Sesame seeds for garnish

Instructions:

1. Heat olive oil in a large skillet or wok over medium heat. Add minced garlic and grated ginger, and cook until fragrant, about 1 minute.
2. Add cubed tofu to the skillet and cook until golden brown on all sides, about 5-7 minutes.
3. Add mixed vegetables to the skillet and stir-fry until tender-crisp, about 5-7 minutes.
4. Stir in soy sauce and sesame oil, and cook for an additional 2 minutes.
5. Serve the stir-fried tofu and vegetables over cooked brown rice, garnished with sesame seeds.

Cooking Time: 15-20 minutes

Nutritional Value (per serving):

- Calories: 300
- Protein: 20g
- Carbohydrates: 30g
- Fat: 12g
- Fiber: 6g

Grilled Chicken Breast with Quinoa Salad

Ingredients:

- 2 boneless, skinless chicken breasts
- 1 cup quinoa, rinsed
- 2 cups water or chicken broth
- 1 cucumber, diced
- 1 tomato, diced
- 1/4 cup chopped fresh parsley
- 1/4 cup feta cheese, crumbled
- 2 tablespoons olive oil
- 1 tablespoon lemon juice
- Salt and pepper to taste

Instructions:

1. Preheat the grill to medium-high heat.
2. Season chicken with salt and pepper. Grill chicken until cooked through, about 6-8 minutes per side.
3. In a saucepan, bring water or chicken broth to a boil. Stir in quinoa, reduce heat to low, cover, and simmer until quinoa is tender and water is absorbed, about 15-20 minutes.
4. In a large bowl, combine cooked quinoa, diced cucumber, diced tomato, chopped parsley, crumbled feta cheese, olive oil,

lemon juice, salt, and pepper. Mix well to combine.

5. Serve grilled chicken breasts with quinoa salad on the side.

Cooking Time: 25-30 minutes

Vegetable and Lentil Soup

Ingredients:

- 1 cup dried lentils, rinsed
- 4 cups vegetable broth
- 2 cups water
- 2 carrots, diced
- 2 celery stalks, diced
- 1 onion, diced
- 2 cloves garlic, minced
- 1 teaspoon dried thyme
- 1 bay leaf
- Salt and pepper to taste
- Fresh parsley for garnish

Instructions:

1. In a large pot, combine dried lentils, vegetable broth, water, diced carrots, diced celery, diced onion, minced garlic, dried thyme, and bay leaf.
2. Bring the soup to a boil, then reduce heat to low and simmer, covered, until lentils

and vegetables are tender, about 30-40 minutes.

3. Season the soup with salt and pepper to taste.
4. Remove the bay leaf from the soup before serving.
5. Garnish each bowl of soup with fresh parsley.

Cooking Time: 40-45 minutes

Poached Cod with Lemon-Dill Sauce

Ingredients:

- 2 cod fillets
- 2 cups vegetable broth
- 1 lemon, thinly sliced
- 2 tablespoons chopped fresh dill
- Salt and pepper to taste
- For the Lemon-Dill Sauce:

- 1/4 cup plain Greek yogurt
- 1 tablespoon lemon juice
- 1 tablespoon chopped fresh dill
- Salt and pepper to taste

Instructions:

1. In a large skillet, bring vegetable broth to a simmer over medium heat.
2. Season cod fillets with salt and pepper, then gently place them in the simmering broth.
3. Arrange lemon slices on top of the cod fillets, then cover and poach until the fish is cooked through and flakes easily with a fork, about 8-10 minutes.
4. While the cod is poaching, prepare the lemon-dill sauce by combining Greek yogurt, lemon juice, chopped dill, salt, and pepper in a small bowl. Mix well to combine.
5. Serve poached cod fillets with lemon-dill sauce drizzled on top, garnished with additional fresh dill.

Cooking Time: 15-20 minutes

Quinoa and Roasted Vegetable Bowl

Ingredients:

- 1 cup quinoa, rinsed
- 2 cups water or vegetable broth
- 2 cups mixed vegetables (such as bell peppers, zucchini, and cherry tomatoes), chopped
- 2 tablespoons olive oil
- 1 teaspoon dried Italian herbs (such as oregano, basil, and thyme)

- Salt and pepper to taste
- 1/4 cup crumbled feta cheese (optional)
- Fresh basil leaves for garnish

Instructions:

1. Preheat the oven to 400°F (200°C).
2. In a saucepan, bring water or vegetable broth to a boil. Stir in quinoa, reduce heat to low, cover, and simmer until quinoa is tender and water is absorbed, about 15-20 minutes.
3. Meanwhile, spread chopped mixed vegetables on a baking sheet lined with parchment paper. Drizzle with olive oil, sprinkle with dried Italian herbs, salt, and pepper, and toss to coat evenly.
4. Roast the vegetables in the preheated oven until tender and lightly browned, about 20-25 minutes, stirring halfway through cooking.
5. To assemble the bowls, divide cooked quinoa among serving bowls and top with roasted vegetables. Sprinkle with crumbled feta cheese (if using) and garnish with fresh basil leaves.
6. Serve hot or at room temperature.

Cooking Time: 35-45 minutes

Baked Chicken and Vegetable Casserole

Ingredients:

- 2 boneless, skinless chicken breasts, diced
- 2 cups mixed vegetables (such as broccoli, carrots, and cauliflower), chopped
- 1 onion, diced
- 2 cloves garlic, minced
- 1 cup chicken broth
- 1/4 cup plain Greek yogurt
- 1 tablespoon olive oil
- 1 teaspoon dried thyme
- Salt and pepper to taste
- 1/4 cup grated Parmesan cheese (optional)

Instructions:

1. Preheat the oven to 375°F (190°C).
2. In a large skillet, heat olive oil over medium heat. Add diced chicken breasts and cook until browned on all sides, about 5-7 minutes. Remove chicken from skillet and set aside.
3. In the same skillet, add diced onion and minced garlic, and cook until softened and fragrant, about 3-4 minutes.
4. Add chopped mixed vegetables to the skillet and cook until slightly tender, about 5 minutes.

5. Return cooked chicken to the skillet and stir in chicken broth, Greek yogurt, dried thyme, salt, and pepper. Mix well to combine.
6. Transfer the chicken and vegetable mixture to a baking dish. Sprinkle grated Parmesan cheese on top (if using).
7. Bake in the preheated oven until bubbly and golden brown, about 25-30 minutes.
8. Serve hot, garnished with fresh herbs if desired.

Cooking Time: 40-45 minutes

Lentil and Vegetable Stir-Fry

Ingredients:

- 1 cup dried green lentils, rinsed
- 2 cups water or vegetable broth
- 2 cups mixed vegetables (such as bell peppers, snap peas, and mushrooms), sliced
- 2 cloves garlic, minced
- 1 tablespoon grated ginger
- 2 tablespoons soy sauce (low-sodium)
- 1 tablespoon sesame oil
- 1 tablespoon olive oil
- Cooked brown rice for serving
- Sesame seeds for garnish

Instructions:

1. In a saucepan, bring water or vegetable broth to a boil. Stir in green lentils, reduce heat to low, cover, and simmer until lentils are tender, about 20-25 minutes.
2. Meanwhile, heat olive oil in a large skillet or wok over medium heat. Add minced garlic and grated ginger, and cook until fragrant, about 1 minute.
3. Add mixed vegetables to the skillet and stir-fry until tender-crisp, about 5-7 minutes.
4. Stir in cooked green lentils, soy sauce, and sesame oil, and cook for an additional 2-3 minutes.
5. Serve the lentil and vegetable stir-fry over cooked brown rice, garnished with sesame seeds.

Cooking Time: 30-35 minutes

Vegetable and Tofu Stir-Fry with Brown Rice
Ingredients:

- 1 block firm tofu, drained and cubed
- 2 cups mixed vegetables (such as broccoli, bell peppers, and carrots), sliced
- 2 cloves garlic, minced
- 1 tablespoon grated ginger
- 2 tablespoons soy sauce (low-sodium)

- 1 tablespoon sesame oil
- 1 tablespoon olive oil
- Cooked brown rice for serving
- Sesame seeds for garnish

Instructions:

1. Heat olive oil in a large skillet or wok over medium heat. Add minced garlic and grated ginger, and cook until fragrant, about 1 minute.
2. Add cubed tofu to the skillet and cook until golden brown on all sides, about 5-7 minutes.
3. Add mixed vegetables to the skillet and stir-fry until tender-crisp, about 5-7 minutes.
4. Stir in soy sauce and sesame oil, and cook for an additional 2-3 minutes.
5. Serve the vegetable and tofu stir-fry over cooked brown rice, garnished with sesame seeds.

Cooking Time: 20-25 minutes

Chapter 7

DESSERT RECIPES SUITABLE FOR A STOMACH ULCER DIET FOR SENIORS

Baked Apples with Cinnamon

Ingredients:

- 4 medium-sized apples (such as Granny Smith or Honey crisp)
- 2 tablespoons honey
- 1 teaspoon ground cinnamon
- 1/4 cup chopped walnuts or almonds (optional)

Instructions:

1. Preheat the oven to 375°F (190°C).
2. Core the apples and place them in a baking dish.
3. Drizzle honey over the apples and sprinkle with cinnamon.
4. If desired, stuff the centers of the apples with chopped nuts.
5. Bake in the preheated oven for 25-30 minutes, or until the apples are tender.
6. Serve warm, optionally topped with a dollop of Greek yogurt or a sprinkle of additional cinnamon.

Cooking time: 25-30 minutes

Nutritional value (per serving):

- Calories: 120
- Protein: 1g
- Fat: 0.5g
- Carbohydrates: 30g
- Fiber: 4g

Chia Seed Pudding with Berries

Ingredients:

- 1/4 cup chia seeds
- 1 cup unsweetened almond milk or coconut milk
- 1 tablespoon honey or maple syrup (optional)
- 1/2 teaspoon vanilla extract
- 1 cup mixed berries (such as strawberries, blueberries, and raspberries)

Instructions:

1. In a bowl, whisk together chia seeds, almond milk, honey or maple syrup (if using), and vanilla extract.
2. Cover and refrigerate for at least 2 hours or overnight, stirring occasionally, until the mixture thickens into a pudding-like consistency.

3. To serve, divide the chia seed pudding into individual serving cups and top with mixed berries.
4. Enjoy chilled.

Cooking time: 2 hours (inactive time)

Nutritional value (per serving):

- Calories: 150
- Protein: 4g
- Fat: 7g
- Carbohydrates: 20g
- Fiber: 10g

Frozen Yogurt Bark

Ingredients:

- 2 cups plain Greek yogurt
- 2 tablespoons honey or maple syrup
- 1/2 teaspoon vanilla extract
- 1/2 cup mixed berries (such as strawberries, blueberries, and raspberries)
- 1/4 cup chopped nuts (such as almonds or walnuts)

Instructions:

1. In a bowl, mix together Greek yogurt, honey or maple syrup, and vanilla extract until well combined.

2. Line a baking sheet with parchment paper.
3. Spread the yogurt mixture evenly onto the parchment paper, about 1/4 inch thick.
4. Sprinkle mixed berries and chopped nuts evenly over the yogurt layer.
5. Place the baking sheet in the freezer and freeze for at least 2 hours, or until the yogurt is firm.
6. Once frozen, break the yogurt bark into pieces and serve immediately.
7. Store any leftovers in an airtight container in the freezer.

Cooking time: 2 hours (inactive time)

Nutritional value (per serving):

- Calories: 120
- Protein: 8g
- Fat: 5g
- Carbohydrates: 12g
- Fiber: 2g

Rice Pudding with Cinnamon

Ingredients:

- 1/2 cup Arborio rice
- 2 cups unsweetened almond milk or coconut milk
- 2 tablespoons honey or maple syrup

- 1 teaspoon vanilla extract
- 1/2 teaspoon ground cinnamon
- Pinch of salt

Instructions:

1. In a saucepan, combine rice, almond milk or coconut milk, honey or maple syrup, vanilla extract, cinnamon, and a pinch of salt.
2. Bring the mixture to a boil over medium heat, then reduce the heat to low and simmer, stirring occasionally, for 20-25 minutes, or until the rice is cooked and the mixture has thickened.
3. Remove from heat and let cool slightly.
4. Serve warm or chilled, sprinkled with additional cinnamon if desired.

Cooking time: 25-30 minutes

Nutritional value (per serving):

- Calories: 180
- Protein: 3g
- Fat: 2g
- Carbohydrates: 35g
- Fiber: 1g

Poached Pears with Ginger

Ingredients:

- 4 ripe but firm pears, peeled and cored
- 2 cups water
- 1/4 cup honey or maple syrup
- 1-inch piece of fresh ginger, thinly sliced
- 1 cinnamon stick
- 1 teaspoon vanilla extract

Instructions:

1. In a large saucepan, combine water, honey or maple syrup, ginger slices, cinnamon stick, and vanilla extract.
2. Bring the mixture to a simmer over medium heat.
3. Add the peeled and cored pears to the saucepan, ensuring they are fully submerged in the liquid.
4. Cover and simmer for 20-25 minutes, or until the pears are tender but not mushy, turning them occasionally to ensure even cooking.
5. Remove the saucepan from heat and let the pears cool in the poaching liquid.
6. Once cooled, remove the pears from the liquid and transfer to serving plates.
7. Optionally, drizzle with a spoonful of the poaching liquid before serving.

Cooking time: 25-30 minutes

Nutritional value (per serving):

- Calories: 140
- Protein: 1g
- Fat: 0g
- Carbohydrates: 35g
- Fiber: 4g

Banana Oatmeal Cookies

Ingredients:

- 2 ripe bananas, mashed
- 1 cup rolled oats
- 1/4 cup chopped nuts (such as walnuts or almonds)
- 1/4 cup dried fruit (such as raisins or cranberries)
- 1 teaspoon ground cinnamon
- 1/2 teaspoon vanilla extract

Instructions:

1. Preheat the oven to 350°F (175°C).
2. In a bowl, combine mashed bananas, rolled oats, chopped nuts, dried fruit, cinnamon, and vanilla extract.
3. Mix until all ingredients are well combined.

4. Drop spoonfuls of the mixture onto a baking sheet lined with parchment paper, pressing down lightly to flatten each cookie.
5. Bake in the preheated oven for 12-15 minutes, or until the cookies are golden brown and set.
6. Remove from the oven and let cool on the baking sheet for 5 minutes before transferring to a wire rack to cool completely.

Cooking time: 12-15 minutes

Nutritional value (per serving, based on 2 cookies):

- Calories: 120
- Protein: 3g
- Fat: 4g
- Carbohydrates: 20g
- Fiber: 3g

Coconut Yogurt Parfait

Ingredients:

- 1 cup unsweetened coconut yogurt
- 1/4 cup granola (look for low-sugar options)

- 1/2 cup mixed berries (such as strawberries, blueberries, and raspberries)
- 1 tablespoon shredded coconut

Instructions:

1. In a serving glass or bowl, layer coconut yogurt, granola, mixed berries, and shredded coconut.
2. Repeat layers until the glass or bowl is filled.
3. Serve immediately, or cover and refrigerate until ready to serve.

Cooking time: None (assembly only)

Nutritional value (per serving):

- Calories: 180
- Protein: 4g
- Fat: 7g
- Carbohydrates: 25g
- Fiber: 5g

Pumpkin Spice Baked Oatmeal Cups

Ingredients:

- 2 cups rolled oats
- 1 teaspoon baking powder
- 1 teaspoon pumpkin pie spice
- 1/4 teaspoon salt
- 1/4 cup honey or maple syrup

- 1 cup unsweetened almond milk or coconut milk
- 1/2 cup pumpkin puree
- 1 egg
- 1 teaspoon vanilla extract
- 1/4 cup chopped nuts (such as pecans or walnuts)

Instructions:

1. Preheat the oven to 350°F (175°C).
2. In a large bowl, combine rolled oats, baking powder, pumpkin pie spice, and salt.
3. In a separate bowl, whisk together honey or maple syrup, almond milk or coconut milk, pumpkin puree, egg, and vanilla extract.
4. Pour the wet ingredients into the dry ingredients and mix until well combined.
5. Fold in chopped nuts.
6. Divide the mixture evenly among a greased muffin tin, filling each cup about 3/4 full.
7. Bake in the preheated oven for 20-25 minutes, or until the tops are golden brown and set.
8. Remove from the oven and let cool in the muffin tin for 5 minutes before transferring to a wire rack to cool completely.

Cooking time: 20-25 minutes

Nutritional value (per serving, based on 1 oatmeal cup):

- Calories: 150
- Protein: 4g
- Fat: 5g
- Carbohydrates: 25g
- Fiber: 3g

Berry Yogurt Popsicles

Ingredients:

- 1 cup plain Greek yogurt
- 1/4 cup honey or maple syrup
- 1 teaspoon vanilla extract
- 1 cup mixed berries (such as strawberries, blueberries, and raspberries)

Instructions:

1. In a blender or food processor, combine Greek yogurt, honey or maple syrup, and vanilla extract. Blend until smooth.
2. Add mixed berries to the yogurt mixture and pulse a few times until the berries are slightly mashed but still chunky.
3. Divide the mixture evenly among popsicle molds.

4. Insert popsicle sticks into the molds and freeze for at least 4 hours, or until the popsicles are frozen solid.
5. To unmold, run warm water over the outside of the molds for a few seconds to loosen the popsicles.
6. Serve immediately and enjoy.

Cooking time: 4 hours (inactive time)

Nutritional value (per serving):

- Calories: 80
- Protein: 3g
- Fat: 1g
- Carbohydrates: 15g
- Fiber: 2g

Almond Butter Banana Bites

Ingredients:

- 2 ripe bananas, peeled and sliced
- 1/4 cup almond butter (or any nut or seed butter of choice)
- 2 tablespoons unsweetened shredded coconut
- 2 tablespoons chopped nuts (such as almonds or walnuts)

Instructions:

1. Spread almond butter on one side of each banana slice.
2. Sprinkle shredded coconut and chopped nuts over the almond butter.
3. Place another banana slice on top to make a sandwich.
4. Repeat with the remaining banana slices.
5. Serve immediately, or refrigerate for 30 minutes to allow the almond butter to firm up slightly.

Cooking time: None

Nutritional value (per serving):

- Calories: 120
- Protein: 3g
- Fat: 8g
- Carbohydrates: 12g
- Fiber: 3g

Chapter 7

SATISFYING SNACKS

1. Fresh Fruit Slices with Cottage Cheese

Ingredients:

- Assorted fresh fruits (e.g., apples, bananas, berries)
- Low-fat cottage cheese

Instructions:

1. Wash and slice the fresh fruits into bite-sized pieces.
2. Serve the fruit slices with a side of low-fat cottage cheese.
3. Enjoy as a refreshing and satisfying snack.

Nutritional Value (per serving):

- Calories: 120
- Protein: 8g
- Carbohydrates: 20g
- Fat: 1g
- Fiber: 3g

2. Hummus with Veggie Sticks

Ingredients:

- Hummus
- Assorted fresh vegetables (e.g., carrots, cucumber, bell peppers)

Instructions:

1. Wash and slice the fresh vegetables into sticks.
2. Serve the veggie sticks with a side of hummus for dipping.
3. Enjoy this crunchy and nutritious snack option.

Nutritional Value (per serving):

- Calories: 150
- Protein: 5g
- Carbohydrates: 15g
- Fat: 8g
- Fiber: 6g

3. Trail Mix with Nuts and Dried Fruits

Ingredients:

- Mixed nuts (e.g., almonds, walnuts, cashews)
- Dried fruits (e.g., raisins, apricots, cranberries)

Instructions:

1. Mix together the mixed nuts and dried fruits in a bowl.
2. Portion out the trail mix into individual servings.
3. Enjoy this convenient and portable snack option.

Nutritional Value (per serving):

- Calories: 200
- Protein: 6g
- Carbohydrates: 20g
- Fat: 12g
- Fiber: 4g

4. Greek Yogurt Parfait

Ingredients:

- Greek yogurt (plain or flavored)
- Fresh berries (e.g., strawberries, blueberries)
- Granola (low-sugar)

Instructions:

1. Layer Greek yogurt, fresh berries, and granola in a serving glass or bowl.
2. Repeat the layers until the glass or bowl is filled.
3. Enjoy this creamy and satisfying parfait.

Nutritional Value (per serving):

- Calories: 180
- Protein: 15g
- Carbohydrates: 25g
- Fat: 5g
- Fiber: 4g

6. Apple Slices with Nut Butter

Ingredients:

- Apples
- Nut butter (e.g., almond butter, peanut butter)

Instructions:

1. Wash and slice the apples into wedges.
2. Spread nut butter onto each apple slice.
3. Enjoy this crunchy and flavorful snack option.

Nutritional Value (per serving):

- Calories: 160
- Protein: 4g
- Carbohydrates: 20g
- Fat: 8g
- Fiber: 5g

5. Cucumber and Tomato Salad

Ingredients:

- Cucumber
- Tomato
- Olive oil
- Lemon juice
- Fresh herbs (e.g., parsley, basil)
- Salt and pepper

Instructions:

1. Wash and dice the cucumber and tomato.
2. Toss the diced cucumber and tomato with olive oil, lemon juice, fresh herbs, salt, and pepper.
3. Chill the salad in the refrigerator before serving.
4. Enjoy this refreshing and hydrating snack option.

Nutritional Value (per serving):

- Calories: 70
- Protein: 1g
- Carbohydrates: 5g
- Fat: 5g
- Fiber: 2g

7. Whole Grain Crackers with Tuna Salad

Ingredients:

- Whole grain crackers
- Canned tuna (in water)
- Greek yogurt
- Celery
- Red onion
- Lemon juice
- Salt and pepper

Instructions:

1. Drain the canned tuna and transfer it to a bowl.
2. Add Greek yogurt, diced celery, diced red onion, lemon juice, salt, and pepper to the bowl.
3. Mix until well combined.
4. Serve the tuna salad with whole grain crackers.
5. Enjoy this protein-rich and satisfying snack option.

Nutritional Value (per serving):

- Calories: 160
- Protein: 15g
- Carbohydrates: 15g
- Fat: 5g
- Fiber: 3g

8. Rice Cake with Avocado Smash

Ingredients:

- Rice cakes (whole grain)
- Avocado
- Lime juice
- Red pepper flakes (optional)
- Salt and pepper

Instructions:

1. Slice the avocado and place it in a bowl.
2. Mash the avocado with a fork and add lime juice, red pepper flakes (if using), salt, and pepper to taste.
3. Spread the avocado smash onto rice cakes.
4. Enjoy this simple and nutritious snack option.

Nutritional Value (per serving):

- Calories: 120
- Protein: 2g
- Carbohydrates: 15g
- Fat: 7g
- Fiber: 4g

9. Boiled Egg with Whole Grain Toast

Ingredients:

- Eggs
- Whole grain bread
- Butter or avocado (optional)
- Salt and pepper

Instructions:

1. Hard-boil the eggs and peel off the shells.
2. Toast the whole grain bread until golden brown.
3. Spread butter or mashed avocado onto the toast (if desired).
4. Slice the boiled eggs and place them on top of the toast.
5. Season with salt and pepper
6. Enjoy this protein-rich and satisfying snack option.

Nutritional Value (per serving):

- Calories: 180
- Protein: 12g
- Carbohydrates: 15g
- Fat: 8g
- Fiber: 3g

10. Chia Seed Pudding with Berries

Ingredients:

- Chia seeds
- Unsweetened almond milk
- Vanilla extract
- Fresh berries (e.g., strawberries, raspberries)
- Honey or maple syrup (optional)

Instructions:

1. In a bowl or jar, mix together chia seeds, almond milk, and vanilla extract.
2. Stir well to combine and let it sit for at least 30 minutes or until thickened.
3. Serve the chia seed pudding with fresh berries on top.
4. Drizzle with honey or maple syrup if desired.
5. Enjoy this nutritious and fiber-rich snack option.

Nutritional Value (per serving):

- Calories: 150
- Protein: 4g
- Carbohydrates: 20g
- Fat: 7g

Chapter 8

FLAVORFUL AND HEALING BEVERAGE RECIPES

1. Ginger Turmeric Tea

Ingredients:

- 1-inch piece of fresh ginger, peeled and sliced
- 1 teaspoon ground turmeric
- 2 cups water
- Honey (optional, to taste)
- Lemon slices (optional, for garnish)

Instructions:

1. In a small saucepan, bring the water to a boil.
2. Add the sliced ginger and ground turmeric to the boiling water.
3. Reduce the heat to low and simmer for 5-10 minutes.
4. Remove from heat and strain the tea into cups.
5. Add honey to taste, if desired, and garnish with lemon slices.
6. Serve hot.

Cooking Time: 10 minutes

Nutritional Value (per serving):

- Calories: 10
- Carbohydrates: 2g
- Fat: 0g
- Protein: 0g
- Fiber: 1g

2. Chamomile Lavender Tea

Ingredients:

- 1 tablespoon dried chamomile flowers
- 1 teaspoon dried lavender flowers
- 2 cups water
- Honey (optional, to taste)

Instructions:

1. In a teapot or heatproof pitcher, combine the chamomile flowers and lavender flowers.
2. Bring the water to a boil and pour it over the flowers.
3. Cover and let steep for 5-10 minutes.
4. Strain the tea into cups and add honey to taste, if desired.
5. Serve hot.

Cooking Time: 10 minutes

Nutritional Value (per serving):

- Calories: 5
- Carbohydrates: 1g
- Fat: 0g
- Protein: 0g
- Fiber: 0g

3. Mint Cucumber Cooler

Ingredients:

- 1 cucumber, peeled and sliced
- 1/4 cup fresh mint leaves
- 2 cups water
- Ice cubes
- Lemon slices (optional, for garnish)

Instructions:

1. In a blender, combine the cucumber slices, mint leaves, and water.
2. Blend until smooth.
3. Strain the mixture to remove any pulp.
4. Pour the cucumber-mint juice over ice cubes in glasses.
5. Garnish with lemon slices, if desired.
6. Serve chilled.

Cooking Time: 5 minutes

Nutritional Value (per serving):

- Calories: 10
- Carbohydrates: 2g
- Fat: 0g
- Protein: 0g
- Fiber: 1g

4. Banana Almond Smoothie

Ingredients:

- 1 ripe banana
- 1 tablespoon almond butter
- 1 cup almond milk
- 1/2 teaspoon ground cinnamon
- Ice cubes (optional)

Instructions:

1. In a blender, combine the ripe banana, almond butter, almond milk, and ground cinnamon.
2. Add ice cubes if desired for a colder smoothie.
3. Blend until smooth and creamy.
4. Pour the smoothie into glasses.
5. Serve immediately.

Cooking Time: 5 minutes

Nutritional Value (per serving):

- Calories: 150
- Carbohydrates: 20g
- Fat: 7g
- Protein: 3g
- Fiber: 3g

5. Papaya Pineapple Smoothie

Ingredients:

- 1 cup ripe papaya, diced
- 1/2 cup fresh pineapple chunks
- 1/2 cup coconut water
- 1 tablespoon honey (optional, to taste)
- Ice cubes (optional)

Instructions:

1. In a blender, combine the diced papaya, pineapple chunks, coconut water, and honey.
2. Add ice cubes if desired for a colder smoothie.
3. Blend until smooth and creamy.
4. Pour the smoothie into glasses.
5. Serve immediately.

Cooking Time: 5 minutes

Nutritional Value (per serving):

- Calories: 100
- Carbohydrates: 25g
- Fat: 0.5g
- Protein: 1g
- Fiber: 3g

6. Aloe Vera Lemonade

Ingredients:

- 1 cup fresh aloe Vera gel (peeled and cubed)
- Juice of 2 lemons
- 3 cups water
- 2 tablespoons honey (optional, to taste)
- Ice cubes
- Lemon slices (optional, for garnish)

Instructions:

1. In a blender, combine the fresh aloe vera gel, lemon juice, water, and honey.
2. Blend until smooth.
3. Strain the mixture to remove any pulp.
4. Pour the aloe Vera lemonade over ice cubes in glasses.
5. Garnish with lemon slices, if desired.
6. Serve chilled.

Cooking Time: 10 minutes

Nutritional Value (per serving):

- Calories: 40
- Carbohydrates: 10g
- Fat: 0g
- Protein: 0g
- Fiber: 1g

7. Carrot Apple Ginger Juice

Ingredients:

- 2 carrots, peeled and chopped
- 1 apple, cored and chopped
- 1-inch piece of fresh ginger, peeled
- 1 cup water
- Ice cubes (optional)

Instructions:

1. In a juicer or blender, combine the chopped carrots, apple, ginger, and water.
2. Blend until smooth.
3. Strain the juice to remove any pulp.
4. Pour the carrot apple ginger juice over ice cubes in glasses.
5. Serve immediately.

Cooking Time: 5 minutes

Nutritional Value (per serving):

- Calories: 60
- Carbohydrates: 15g
- Fat: 0g
- Protein: 1g
- Fiber: 3g

8. Berry Spinach Smoothie

Ingredients:

- 1/2 cup mixed berries (such as strawberries, blueberries, raspberries)
- 1 cup fresh spinach leaves
- 1/2 cup Greek yogurt
- 1 tablespoon honey (optional, to taste)
- Ice cubes (optional)

Instructions:

1. In a blender, combine the mixed berries, spinach leaves, Greek yogurt, and honey.
2. Add ice cubes if desired for a colder smoothie.
3. Blend until smooth and creamy.
4. Pour the smoothie into glasses.
5. Serve immediately.

Cooking Time: 5 minutes

Nutritional Value (per serving):

- Calories: 80
- Carbohydrates: 15g
- Fat: 0g
- Protein: 5g
- Fiber: 3g

9. Peppermint Green Tea

Ingredients:

- 2 green tea bags
- 1 tablespoon fresh peppermint leaves
- 2 cups water
- Honey (optional, to taste)
- Lemon slices (optional, for garnish)

Instructions:

1. In a teapot, steep the green tea bags and peppermint leaves in hot water for 3-5 minutes.
2. Remove the tea bags and peppermint leaves.
3. Add honey to taste, if desired.
4. Garnish with lemon slices, if desired.
5. Serve hot.

Cooking Time: 5 minutes

Nutritional Value (per serving):

- Calories: 5
- Carbohydrates: 1g
- Fat: 0g
- Protein: 0g
- Fiber: 0g

10. Coconut Water Kefir

Ingredients:

- 2 cups coconut water
- 2 tablespoons kefir grains
- 1 tablespoon honey (optional, to taste)

Instructions:

1. In a clean glass jar, combine the coconut water and kefir grains.
2. Cover the jar with a clean cloth and secure with a rubber band.
3. Let the mixture ferment at room temperature for 24-48 hours, depending on desired tartness.
4. Once fermented, strain the kefir grains from the coconut water.
5. Stir in honey to taste, if desired.
6. Transfer the coconut water kefir to a sealed container and refrigerate until chilled.
7. Serve cold.

Cooking Time: 24-48 hours (fermentation time)

Nutritional Value (per serving):

- Calories: 50
- Carbohydrates: 12g
- Fat: 0g
- Protein: 0g
- Fiber: 0g

Chapter 10

TIPS FOR DINING OUT:

Dining out can be enjoyable and convenient, but it can also present challenges for individuals with stomach ulcers. Making healthy choices at restaurants, managing portion sizes, and communicating dietary needs are essential strategies for seniors to maintain their stomach ulcer diet while dining out.

Making Healthy Choices at Restaurants:

1. Review the menu in advance: Many restaurants now provide their menus online, allowing you to review options before arriving. Look for dishes that are lower in fat, spice, and acidity, and avoid items known to trigger stomach ulcer symptoms.

2. Choose simple, grilled options: Go for grilled or baked proteins such as chicken, fish, or tofu, and request sauces and dressings on the side to control portion sizes and avoid excess fat.

3. Select steamed or lightly cooked vegetables: Steamed or lightly cooked vegetables are gentler on the stomach and provide essential nutrients without added fat or seasoning.

4. Ask for modifications: Don't hesitate to ask your server for modifications to accommodate your dietary needs. Requesting substitutions or omissions can help ensure that your meal is stomach ulcer-friendly.

5. Be cautious with appetizers and sides: Be mindful of appetizers and side dishes that may contain ingredients known to trigger stomach ulcer symptoms, such as spicy sauces or fried foods. Opt for simpler options like salads or steamed vegetables when available.

Managing Portion Sizes:

1. Split entrees or ask for a half portion: Restaurant portion sizes are often larger than what is necessary for a single meal. Consider sharing an entree with a dining companion or asking for a half portion to avoid overeating.

2. Request a to-go box: If your meal is served in a large portion, ask your server for a to-go box at the beginning of the meal. Portion out a suitable amount for your meal and set aside the rest to enjoy later.

3. Focus on mindful eating: Pay attention to hunger and fullness cues throughout your meal and stop eating when you feel satisfied. Avoid rushing through your meal and take time to savor each bite.

Communicating Dietary Needs:

1. Inform your server of your dietary restrictions: When dining out, don't hesitate to inform your server of your dietary needs, including any food allergies or intolerances. Be clear about what you can and cannot eat to ensure that your meal is prepared accordingly.

2. Ask questions about preparation methods: If you're unsure about how a dish is prepared or the ingredients used, don't hesitate to ask your server for more information. Inquire about cooking methods, seasonings, and potential substitutions.

3. Be polite and appreciative: Remember that restaurant staffs are there to help accommodate your needs. Be polite and appreciative of their efforts to make your dining experience enjoyable and stomach ulcer-friendly.

ADDITIONAL RESOURCES AND SUPPORT

Support Groups and Communities:

1. American Gastroenterological Association (AGA): The AGA offers resources and support for individuals living with gastrointestinal conditions, including stomach ulcers. Their website provides access to educational materials, webinars, and information on local support groups.

2. Health Boards (www.healthboards.com): Health Boards is an online community where individuals can connect with others facing similar health challenges, including stomach ulcers. The platform features discussion forums, support groups, and user-generated content related to digestive health.

3. Local Hospitals and Medical Centers: Many hospitals and medical centers host support groups or educational events for individuals living with digestive disorders. Reach out to your healthcare provider or local hospital to inquire about available resources and opportunities to connect with others in your community.

4. Meetup.com: Meetup.com is a platform that facilitates in-person gatherings and events based on shared interests and hobbies. Users can search for groups related to digestive health or stomach ulcers in their area and join meetings or activities to connect with peers facing similar challenges.

5. Online Forums and Social Media Groups: There are numerous online forums and social media groups dedicated to digestive health and stomach ulcer support. Platforms like Facebook, Reddit, and Inspire host communities where individuals can ask questions, share experiences, and find support from others navigating similar health journeys.

By exploring these additional resources and support options, seniors managing stomach ulcers can access valuable information, connect with peers, and find encouragement on their path to improved digestive health and overall well-being. Whether through online resources, educational materials, or community engagement, individuals can find the support they need to effectively manage their condition and live life to the fullest.

Conclusion:

Managing stomach ulcers can be a challenging journey, but with the right knowledge, resources, and support, seniors can effectively navigate their condition and improve their quality of life. Throughout this guide, we've explored the importance of dietary choices, lifestyle modifications, and self-care strategies for individuals living with stomach ulcers. By adopting a stomach ulcer-friendly diet, making healthy lifestyle choices, and seeking support from healthcare professionals and peers, seniors can alleviate symptoms, promote healing, and prevent recurrence of ulcers.

As we conclude this book, it's essential to emphasize the importance of patience and persistence in managing stomach ulcers. Healing takes time, and setbacks may occur along the way. However, with dedication, perseverance, and the support of healthcare professionals and loved ones, seniors can overcome the challenges posed by stomach ulcers and lead fulfilling lives.

Cheers to your health!

Thank you for embarking on this journey. Your commitment to health and well-being inspires me. May these recipes nourish your body, delight your palate, and bring relief.

Cheers to your continued wellness.

www.ingramcontent.com/pod-product-compliance
Lightning Source LLC
Chambersburg PA
CBHW071058290526
45795CB00004B/1548